DIY Shampoo:

25 Best Organic Homemade Shampoo Recipes

Table of content

Introduction

Every person in the world uses shampoo of some description. It is designed to help you stay clean and can also help you to smell nice. Remaining clean is important as it will reduce the chance of infections and diseases, especially if you have cut or injured yourself. Shampooing can also help the body to remove the top layer of dead cells which can otherwise cause itching and even skin issues.

If you enter any beauty shop you will see a huge range of different shampoos; each one smells differently and may promise different things, or be designed to treat certain types of hair. Yet, despite this array of fantastic products more and more people are turning to a more natural approach; DIY shampoo. In fact, this is how the original shampoos were made and there is some benefit to knowing exactly what has been included in your shampoo.

Shampoo was originally invented as long ago as the early part of the 1500's. It appears to have been first used in India where the locals used the pulp of a fruit which was called soapberries. This was merged with hibiscus flowers and herbs to create a shampoo for washing their hair. The increase in trade between India and England saw the introduction of this new product to the market. Of course, at first it was extremely expensive and only available to the nobility or professional hair stylists. At this point shampoo would have only been available in a similar format to a bar of soap.

By the 1800's shampoo had made it into the majority of households although it was still used sparingly. It was until the early part of the twentieth century that the New York Times recommended using shampoo on your hair at least once every couple of weeks. This led to the development of liquid shampoo in the 1920's; something which dramatically changed availability and the usage patterns of many people. In modern times the general consensus is to wash your hair two or three times a week; however there are many people who enjoy the sensation of clean hair so much that they do it every day.

Over the last hundred years shampoos have developed dramatically and the ingredients have been adjusted to provide the perfect wash and shine. You hair should look and feel clean as well as being clean. Modern products work hard to balance the need to strip away environmental dirt and natural oils and skin without removing the good stuff your body and hair need. However it is a careful balancing act which is often different from person to person. It has led to an array of different types of shampoo ranging from gentle and bay friendly to animal shampoos. But, despite the advances there are still people who believe that they will have a more natural and better looking hair by returning to the old methods. These people still shampoo their hair, but they create their own shampoos from a mixture of ingredients which are designed to produce the right result. The following pages will illustrate some of the most popular recipes.

Chapter 1 – 10 Basic Shampoo Recipes to get you Started

There are a range of arguments regarding why shampoo is necessary. Many people may point to the fact that they have not used shampoo in a year or that it used to be the norm not to shampoo and everyone didn't suddenly develop greasy hair. In fact the modern way of life means that many people adds styling products to their hair and it is these which need to be washed off properly. In theory, simple washing your hair in water will clean it, however, it is unlikely to remove all the styling products, particularly items such as hair gel.

In order to combat this and resist the need to spend copious amounts of funds on an array of beauty products it has become increasingly common for people to adopt one of the following basic shampooing recipes:

1. *Simply Shampoo*

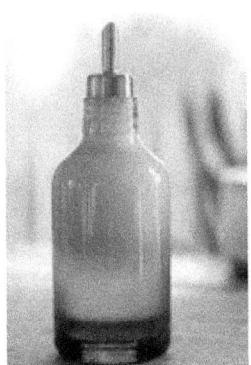

This is one of the simplest methods of making shampoo. Simply add ¼ cup of coconut milk to ¼ cup liquid castile soap and twenty drops of your choice of essential oils. You can also add half a teaspoon of olive oil to help if you naturally have dry hair. This should all be mixed in an old shampoo bottle; you need to ensure you shake the bottle very well and then put it in your shower tray ready for use. It is recommended to discard any still in the bottle after a month. You will also need to give the bottle a good shake before you use it; it is recommended you use just one teaspoon full each time you need to shampoo; whether this is daily or weekly.

2. *Stinging Nettle Shampoo*

To create this unusual concoction you will need 500ml of organic nettle shampoo; two tablespoons of Panthenol solution, 25ml of stinging nettle extract; 50ml of castor oil and three vials of vitamin B Complex.

You can then combine all the ingredients into one glass jar; this shampoo is said to help reduce thinning of your hair and will improve the overall condition of your hair. You should see a dramatic improvement within four to six weeks. However, it is worth noting that the Panthenol coats the hair making it feel stiffer but protecting it at the same time. It is advisable to use a clarifying treatment regularly to ensure the Panthenol is kept in balance. It is also very effective at reducing oiliness in your hair which is of particular benefit if you suffer from this issue.

3. Baking Soda Shampoo

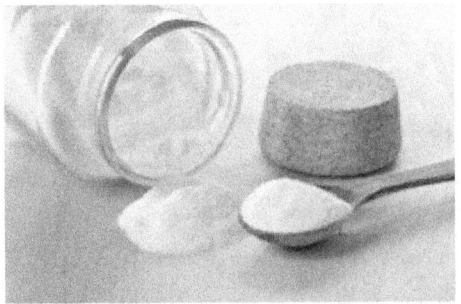

This shampoo has been designed to help with removing excess sebum and reducing any build up of dandruff. People who use this have testified to the fact it can keep your hair looking and feeling clean for several days; in fact they often end up washing it as they feel they ought to and not because they actually need to.

Creating the shampoo is incredibly simple. You will need one tablespoon of baking soda and either a cup of water for a strong solution or two cups for a weaker solution. You can then add it to your hair when washing, just as you would if using a regular shampoo. It is best to spend a few minute massaging it into your scalp to ensure it has the best possible effect and give it a few minutes to work; you will be surprised at how effective the results are.

4. Cucumber & Lemon Shampoo

You are almost certainly aware of the power of lemons already. They have been used throughout history to help clean a variety of surfaces and even to write or read invisible messages. Cucumbers have also developed a reputation as an excellent way of nourishing your body and skin in particular. Mix the two together and you have a potent solution for dry scalp or a quick and easy way to achieve fresh smelling and clean looking hair.

To make this shampoo you simply need to peel a lemon and place the lemon in a food processor. You will then need to peel a cucumber and add that to the food processor. Simply turn the processor on and wait until you have a paste; it should be smooth; although there will always be some bits in it. This paste can then be lathered into your hair to clean and nourish it. You will need to be certain that you are massaging it in really well before you take as much care rinsing it off. You will have lots of bits of lemon in your hair so thorough rinsing is essential. The results will be visible almost immediately.

5. Cornstarch Shampoo

This is a surprisingly effective and cheap solution to your hair care issues. It costs a fraction of the amount a bottle of shampoo does and can be made in a few moments. It is an excellent way to treat oily hair; starting with the roots.

To use this version of shampoo you simply buy a packet of cornstarch. You can then apply this to your roots whenever they start to look oily or even at set intervals. It is best to dab the powder directly onto your hair and roots using a cloth or brush. You will then need to wait for a few minutes before you brush the powder out and your treatment is complete!

You can also adapt this powder to help thicken your hair. Simply add a tablespoon of baking soda to a cup of water and a tablespoon of cornstarch. This will increase the volume and thickness of your hair.

6. Dry Hair

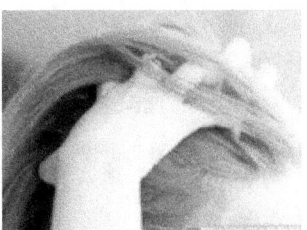

Anyone who suffers from dry hair will appreciate the difficulty in finding the right treatment for your hair and scalp. There are hundreds of products which promise to help with the issue but usually only offer temporary relief. Fortunately there is a natural alternative which has been used for many years and acts as both a shampoo and a conditioner. It is easy and cheap to make; meaning that anyone can try this method.

You will simply need to mix one cup of liquid organic Castile soap with two tablespoons of apple cider vinegar, one tablespoon of Tea Tree Oil and a quarter of a cup of water.

Mix them thoroughly and then pour into a spray bottle, you can also add a few drops of your favorite essential oils to improve the scent. Give the bottle a shake before you use it and apply it as you would any other shampoo product.

7. *Coconut Shampoo*

Coconut, or in particularly coconut milk has been used in a huge range of health and beauty products. It is good to eat but also appears to be a valuable addition to many products which promise to soften or beautify your skin. This shampoo is exceptionally good at relieving the problem of dry hair which can cause itchy scalps.

You will need to mix several ingredients together in a suitable container; use a quarter cup coconut milk, a third of a cup of extra mild organic shampoo, one tablespoon of almond oil and your own choice of essential oils; up to ten drops.

Once you have mixed them thoroughly you should also shake them well. It is best to create the shampoo in the bottle you will be using to store and access the shampoo; there is little point in using a second container. You can now use it as you would normal shampoo.

8. Swimming Shampoo

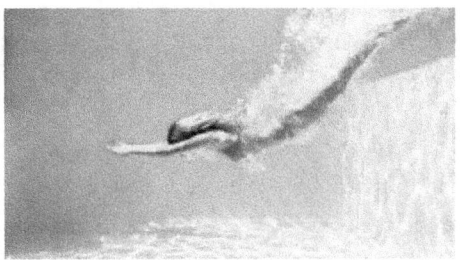

If you are a regular swimmer you will understand the frustration associated with the levels of chlorine in the pool. This can leave your hair dry, damaged and even brittle. Shampooing everyday can make your hair feel better but may not actually improve the quality of your hair. It can also be an issue if you have already dyed your hair, blond hair will often start to go green if you swim regularly.

Fortunately there is an alternative, this DIY shampoo can be used once a week to combat the effects of the pool and can even be used alongside your other shampoos; if you are not willing to give them up at this stage.

You will need to put one liter of water in a pan and bring it to the boil; alternatively you can do it in your kettle if it is large enough. Then pour the boiling water over 120 grams of Castile flakes and stir thoroughly. You can then leave the mixture to cool; once this has happened you can add quarter of a cup of avocado oil. You can also use almond oil or olive oil. Mix the oil in thoroughly before pouring it into your chosen bottle. It is then ready to use and can be applied as per normal shampoo. You will be impressed at the difference it makes.

9. *Anti-Dandruff Shampoo*

There is a huge market full of anti-dandruff shampoos; many of them will offer temporary relief whilst others appear to have no effect at all. In fact it can be very frustrating trying to locate the right product for your needs. Fortunately there is a natural alternative which has proven to be very successful at removing and preventing dandruff.

You will need to start by adding the following ingredients into your food processor; quarter cup of Castile soap liquid, half a cup of grape seed oil and a tablespoon of cider vinegar. On top of this you will need to add three tablespoons of fresh apple juice and six garlic cloves which have been pressed fine.

Once all the ingredients have been added, you can blend them in your food processor until they are smooth. It will then be ready to use. The paste will need to be transferred to a suitable container and should be used within a month of creating it. The effects will be noticeable within a few days.

10.*The Shine Booster*

There are times when you simply want your hair to be shiny; it should look like you have just left the hairdressers. However, despite the promises made on many shampoo product labels, it seems to be a difficult goal to accomplish. You will be pleased to discover there is a natural alternative which can give you the shine you want in next to no time and at very little cost!

To create this you will need to boil one cup of distilled water. Once it has started to boil you should pour it over two tablespoons of dried Rosemary leaves. Leave the mixture to infuse until it is cooled but still warm. You can then strain this to remove the Rosemary. The liquid can then be put in a bowl and you will need to add a quarter cup of Castile liquid soap, two tablespoons of almond oil and half a teaspoon of essential lemon oil. Once you have mixed all these ingredients together you can pour them into a bottle and give them a final shake. Then store in your bathroom where you will remember to use it; preferably shaking the bottle before each use.

Chapter 2 – Another 10 Easily Created Shampoo Recipes

It is difficult to limit the number of possibilities regarding shampoo recipes. There are thousands of combinations; some of which will work well for you and some which will not. This is simply human nature, no two people are the same and the same treatment will not have the same effect on everyone. However, once you have worked out one shampoo recipe which will work for you then it is possible to adapt others which use similar ingredients. In fact, many recipes can be adjusted by simply adding a few drops of your favorite essence. Although this will not change the affect on your hair it will make sure it smells the way you like it.

The following ten recipes can be used by almost anyone to wash your hair without needing expensive shampoo:

1. *Lemon and Aloe Vera Shampoo*

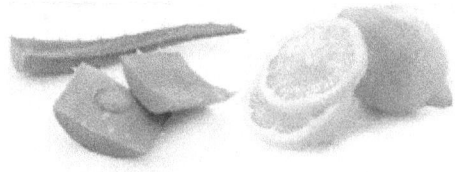

http://www.beinggirlish.com/wp-content/uploads/2016/04/lemon-alovera.jpg

You have probably already come across Aloe Vera; it is used in a variety of beauty treatments as well as an array of health care and medicinal items. It is known to sooth and cool as well as provide valuable nutrients to anyone who needs it. It is also frequently added to many expensive shampoos and body lotions. Fortunately there is a way of creating this shampoo without having to pay the expensive price tags; it is especially effective when dealing with oily hair.

The simplest way of creating your own Aloe Vera shampoo is to mix half a cup of Castile liquid soap with a teaspoon of Aloe Vera gel and two tablespoons of freshly squeezed lemon juice. The whole concoction can be mixed in minutes and is ready to use immediately, it can also be stored in a standard bottle for future use.

2. *Apple Cider Shampoo*

This shampoo is actually made from Apple cider vinegar and it has been shown to be excellent at cleaning your hair thoroughly, even when it has a waxy, dirty feel which is so often a result of the environment you work and live in.

This recipe will allow you to create a shampoo which will cleanse your hair and scalp and leave you feeling fantastic. It is also excellent for nurturing your hair and will leave it soft to the touch.

This is especially useful when first switching from chemical heavy shampoos to either DIY ones or going without shampoo at all; also known as 'no poo'.

The recipe is simple; it requires one egg and two tablespoons of fresh lemon juice. This should go into a food processor along with one teaspoon of apple cider vinegar and 30ml of olive oil. You can then turn your processor on and let it run for several minutes until the mixture is smooth. To use, simply massage it into your scalp and your hair. After a few minutes of rubbing to ensure it has been absorbed by your hair simply wash it out with lukewarm water. You can then bottle it to use immediately.

3. Avocado Shampoo

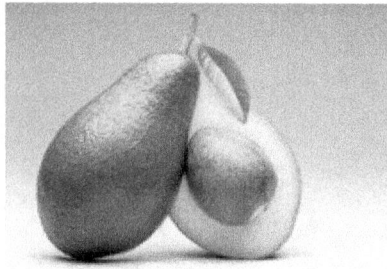

This is an adaption on the basic baking soda shampoo. In fact baking soda can be mixed with a huge array of other ingredients to create a perfectly satisfactory shampoo. Unfortunately to identify the right one could be a long period of trial and error. To avoid this you could try the following recipe. This shampoo is designed to reduce and prevent oily roots whilst providing valuable nutrition for your hair which will ensure it remains healthy and has a natural glow.

You will need one ripe avocado, two teaspoons of baking powder and a quarter cup of water. It is best if the water is distilled but if this is not possible then tap water will suffice.

You can blend these ingredients by hand although it is much easier to use an electronic blender. Once you have created a smooth paste you will be able to bottle it and then use it immediately on your hair. The results will be noticeable in a very short space of time.

4. Egg shampoo

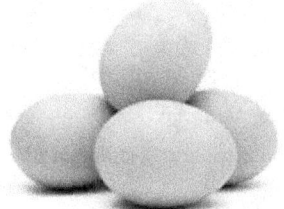

It has been known for many years that eggs are more than just delicious, protein and carbohydrate rich food sources. The same protein can be used in a variety of skin care products to help create the perfect skin, or perfect scalp. It is also an exceptionally good shampoo for keeping your hair moist.

The ingredients are simple; you will need two eggs, three teaspoons of baking powder and two teaspoons of olive oil, alongside this you will also need two teaspoons of lemon juice. You will need to start by beating the two eggs, then slowly add the other ingredients stirring carefully all the time. Once you have created a smooth mixture you will be able to put it in a suitable sized container and use it when needed. It is best to rub your scalp with it gently when you use it to get the best results.

5. *Shikakai and Soap Nut*

This shampoo uses ingredients which have proved to be exceptionally popular in a wide variety of alternative medicines. In fact, these ingredients have also appeared in several mainstream skin and hair care products.

The soap nut has a natural ability to act as an anti-inflammatory and even as an anti-microbial. The traditional Indian medicine of the Shikakai is also known to have the same healing properties. Put together they can make an excellent combination. You will need 100g of soap nuts and two teaspoons of shikakai powder.

To create this shampoo you will need to leave the soap nuts in a bowl of water overnight. In the morning you will be able to place the contents of your bowl into an electric blender and add the requested amount of Shikakai powder. You can then blend the mixture until it is completely smooth. It can then be bottled or used immediately to create healthy looking and feeling hair.

6. The Indian herbal Shampoo

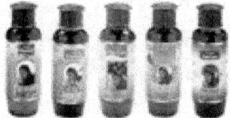

This is a completely natural recipe which, unsurprisingly, originates in India. In fact it will help to restore your natural glow and ensure your hair does not just look and feel healthy; it actually will be.

To create this shampoo you will need 500g of Shikakai, 250g of Fenugreek, 250g of Mung beans, also known as greem gram. Alongside this you will need to find one bunch of curry leaves and one of Basil or Tulsi as well as 100g of soap beans.

All the ingredients should be laid out on a cloth or paper and then can be placed outside the front door to dry in the sunshine. If you leave it in the sun it should be dried within twelve hours, simply leaving it on a cloth on the side, will also take approximately two days. It is best to purchase as many of the ingredients as fresh as possible; this will improve their flavor and the end product. However, you need to note that all your ingredients will need to be dried so you may prefer to purchase dried ones in the first place. If you do have fresh ingredients it is best to grind them up and store them in a glass jar. Ideally you should wait several weeks before starting to make shampoo from this concoction.

You can then remove as much of the dried powder as you need each time you wish to shampoo your hair. Simply mix it with a little water and massage it directly into your scalp. The effects will be obvious after just a few uses.

7. Honey Shampoo

Honey is nature's sweetener. It can be added to almost anything to sweeten it and make it more palatable. It is generally acknowledged to have a huge range of health benefits and is often added to alternative medicine and even some of the mainstream medicines. Of course, it is far too sticky to simply put straight on your hair. Instead, you will need to mix two tablespoons of honey with six tablespoons of warm water and any essential oils you wish to have included to improve the scent.

The water and honey mix should be heated slowly until they are just melting. You will need to stir them to make sure they merge as one. The final mixture will be runny but it can be used on your hair straight away. The shampoo can also be added into your bathroom ready for the next time you shower.

8. Herbal Shampoo

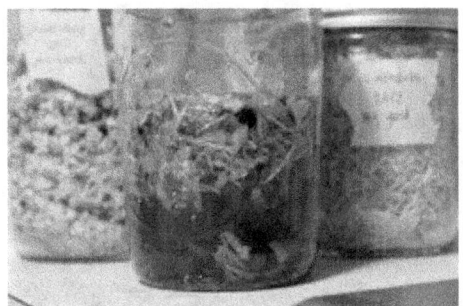

Castile liquid soap is an excellent base for a wide variety of different DIY shampoos; it is readily available and natural. However, if you are looking for a little something more then you should consider creating your own herbal shampoo. It will nourish your hair and leave it looking shiny and feeling great.

It is very easy to make and all the ingredients are natural. Simply place one cup of distilled water into a saucepan and put it on the stove. While you are waiting for it to bowl you can mix as many herbs as you like together to create half a cup of herbs. Alternatively you can use dried flowers. You can choose which herbs or flowers to use according to your own preferences. The herbs should be placed in a sieve which is then placed in the pan of boiling water. You should leave the herbs there for at least thirty minutes; there is no maximum time limit.

You will then need to place a quarter of a cup of Castile liquid soap into a glass jar and add the water, not the herbs. Gently swirl the mixture until it is thoroughly mixed. You can then put your shampoo into a bottle that can be taken into the shower and used easily. Then simply use it as you would normal shampoo; just remember it will be a little runnier.

9. *The Raw Egg Shampoo*

This shampoo is as simple as its name suggests. You take one or two eggs, depending upon the amount of hair you have. Then you beat the eggs and pour them onto top of your head. Eggs are full of protein and this is quickly absorbed by your hair follicles making them stronger and healthier. In fact, they will even make your hair appear to glow as the natural shine is returned.

The beaten egg should be left on for approximately five minutes; you may wish to stand in the shower whilst waiting as it is quite messy and does smell. You may also be surprised by how much of the egg is absorbed into your hair. Once your time is up, simply rinse your hair thoroughly. You may wish to include an apple cider vinegar rinse as previously described.

10.Beer Shampoo

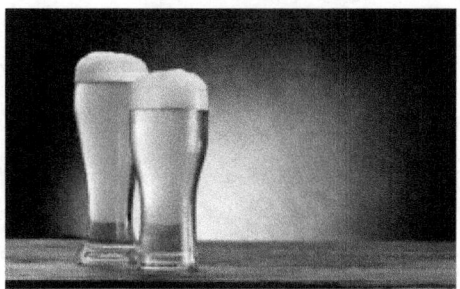

This is a surprising option to many but beer is actually full of proteins which can repair damaged hair and return a natural shine to all your hair. It is even rumored to help prevent hair loss.

You should use beer which is at room temperature and is flat. Ideally it should have been opened and left on the side for two days. It is best to apply it after you have washed your hair with a natural shampoo; the, simply massage it into your hair and leave for several minutes before washing it off.

Chapter 3 – 5 Additional Intriguing Shampoo solutions

It should now be obvious that shampoo can be created out of almost anything; in fact, beer and eggs demonstrate that some shampoos do not even need a recipe; just simply apply a natural product and watch for impressive results.

The following recipes may give you the final inspiration you need to try some of these homemade shampoos:

1. **Milk and Honey**

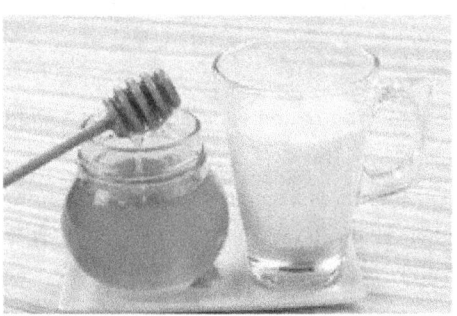

Simply blend two tablespoons of honey with a quarter of a cup of milk. These two healthy foods combine to provide an efficient cleanser, conditioner and moisturizer.

2. Dry Shampoo

This may not be a concept you are particularly familiar with, but it is possible to wash your hair properly without using any water or getting your hair wet. An instant pick you up for your hair can be achieved by sprinkling your scalp with oatmeal and leaving it on for a few minutes. It will absorb excess oil on your scalp and in your roots. After a few minutes brush t carefully out; you will be impressed at how good your hair looks!

You can even add some essential oils to help give your hair a pleasant natural scent.

3. Deep cleaning Sugar

This is more than just a shampoo it is a method of deep cleaning your scalp and thereby providing healthy, thicker and stronger looking hair. Simply ass two tablespoons of brown sugar to a bowl with two tablespoons of finely ground oatmeal and two tablespoons of hair conditioner. Mix the ingredients thoroughly and then have them ready when you shower. You should shampoo your hair first with your chosen natural shampoo and then scrub this concoction into your scalp, working slowly and carefully to ensure you cover your whole scalp.

After the mixture has been on for a few moments simply wash it off.

4. Salt & Olive Oil scrub

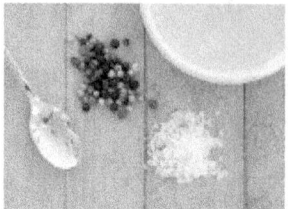

An alternative version of the scalp deep cleanse can be made using two table-spoons of sea salt, two tablespoons of lemon juice and two tablespoons of olive oil. Mix the ingredients thoroughly and then massage into your scalp before you shampoo. After the mixture has been in for a few minutes rinse out and use your regular shampoo.

5. The shampoo bar

The shampoo bar is very similar to an ordinary bar of soap. It is as solid bar which is similar to the original version of shampoo. You can buy a shampoo bar in a shop or you can create your own by mixing Castile liquid soap with your chosen essential oil and adding something such as sand or even oatmeal to act as an exfoliating; effectively scrubbing your scalp whilst providing natural nutrients.

Conclusion

There has been a large amount of publicity in recent years regarding the idea of not using shampoo on your hair. It is a decision which is being made as a reaction to the number of potential dangerous chemicals in modern cleaning and health products. People who advocate the 'no poo' approach are generally trying to minimize their exposure to chemicals which are the body is not naturally exposed to. In effect it is intending to keep the body healthier by remaining closer to nature. It can also be a cheaper way of maintaining your hair.

Many of these people simply wash their hair under cold water and it remains clean and healthy looking. However, this does not work for everyone; either their hair type needs more than just water or they need to feel they are washing it with something to feel clean. The solution to this is outlined in this book, natural shampoo, which can be made at home from natural ingredients. As you will be making the shampoo yourself you will be in control of which ingredients are included and can ensure your body is not exposed to any chemicals or substances which you believe may be harmful or detrimental; whether in the short or long term.

As this book demonstrates, there are an abundance of alternative recipes which can be employed and all of them use readily available ingredients. Although it may take a little trial and error to establish the right DIY shampoos for your needs it is worth experimenting. With a little patience you can create one which has all the benefits of the professional, top class shampoos but without the chemicals and the price tag.

Creating your own shampoo can also be fun! It will enable you to create gifts for others and talk to them about your discoveries; indeed there are several online forums where you can swap ideas and inspiration. Whatever your choice it is important to remember that, providing you are happy with your choice of shampoo and comfortable with the way your hair looks, then the decision you have made regarding the type of shampoo you use is the right one. There is no definitive solution which fits everyone; you must make the right decision for your own needs and lifestyle. But, whether you wish to continue with brand named shampoos or not, you have nothing to lose by trying the recipes in this book.

FREE Bonus Reminder

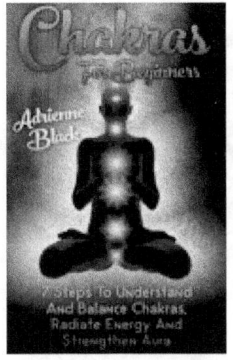

If you have not grabbed it yet, please go ahead and download your special bonus E book *"Chakras for Beginners. 7 Steps To Understand And Balance Chakras, Radiate Energy, And Strengthen Aura"*.

Simply Click the Button Below

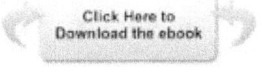

OR Go to This Page

http://lifehacksworld.com/free

BONUS #2: More Free & Discounted Books & Products

Do you want to receive more Free/Discounted Books or Products?

We have a mailing list where we send out our new Books or Products when they go free or with a discount on Amazon. Click on the link below to sign up for Free & Discount Book & Product Promotions.

=> **Sign Up for Free & Discount Book & Product Promotions** <=

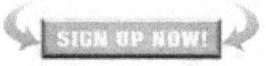

OR Go to this URL

http://zbit.ly/1WBb1Ek

www.ingramcontent.com/pod-product-compliance
Lightning Source LLC
Chambersburg PA
CBHW061946280526
45787CB00004B/1743